GASTRITIS

DIET COOKBOOK FOR BEGINNERS

"A Beginner's Guide to Healing Gastritis Through Wholesome Cooking"

Anita F. MS RDN McCluskey

<u>Disclaimer</u>

The recipes and information provided in this gastritis cookbook for Kids are intended for educational and informational purposes only. It is not a substitute for professional medical advice, diagnosis, or treatment. Always seek the advice of your physician or other qualified health provider with any questions you may have regarding a medical condition. The author and publisher of this cookbook are not liable for any adverse effects or consequences resulting from the use of the information or recipes contained herein."

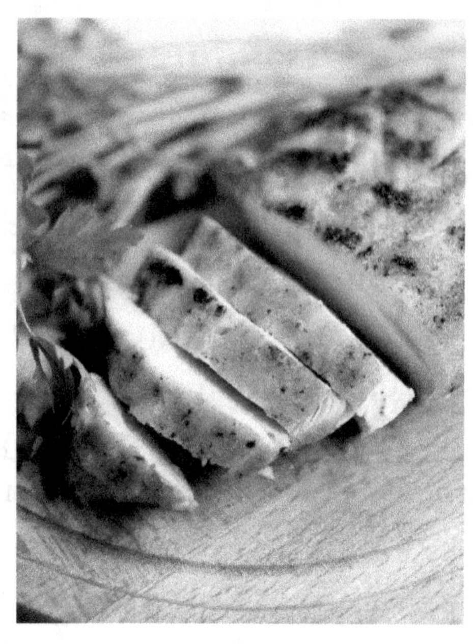

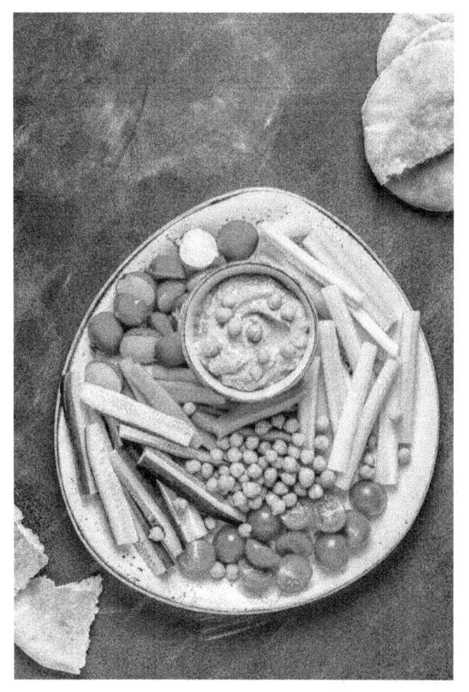

The Ultimate Guide: From Beginner to Grandmaster in Gastritis Diet Cooking

Welcome to the ultimate guide for mastering the art of cooking for gastritis. Whether you're a beginner looking to improve your culinary skills or aiming to become a grandmaster in gastritis diet cooking, this comprehensive guide will provide you with everything you need to know to achieve your goals.

Understanding Gastritis and its Dietary Requirements:

- What is gastritis?
- Symptoms and causes of gastritis
- Importance of diet in managing gastritis
- Foods to avoid and foods to include in a gastritis diet

Getting Started with Gastritis Diet Cooking:

- Essential kitchen tools and equipment
- Stocking your pantry with gastritis-friendly ingredients
- Basic cooking techniques for gastritis-friendly meals
- Meal planning and prepping tips for gastritis diet

<u>*Exploring Gastritis Diet Recipes for Beginners:*</u>

- Simple and delicious recipes suitable for beginners
- Breakfast, lunch, dinner, and snack options
- Tips for flavor enhancement without triggering gastritis symptoms
- Recipe modification for specific dietary restrictions (e.g., gluten-free, dairy-free)

<u>*Advanced Techniques and Culinary Skills:*</u>

- Building flavor profiles in gastritis-friendly dishes
- Incorporating herbs and spices for added taste and health benefits
- Experimenting with different cooking methods (e.g., grilling, roasting, steaming)
- Presentation tips to elevate your gastritis diet meals

Special Hacks for Becoming a Highly Skilled Grandmaster:

Developing your palate:
- tasting and adjusting flavors
- Mastering the art of meal balancing for optimal nutrition
- Creating your gastritis diet recipes
- Incorporating gastritis-friendly cooking into social gatherings and events

Troubleshooting and Adapting to Challenges:
- Dealing with cravings and temptations
- Managing gastritis symptoms during travel and dining out
- Adapting recipes to fit seasonal produce and availability
- Overcoming cooking setbacks and learning from mistakes

Conclusion:

Congratulations on embarking on your journey to becoming a gastritis diet-cooking grandmaster! With dedication, practice, and the knowledge gained from this guide, you'll be able to create delicious and nutritious meals that support your health and well-being. Remember to listen to your body, stay curious, and enjoy the process of cooking and eating mindfully. Happy cooking!

PREFACE

Welcome to the "Gastritis Diet Cookbook for Beginners"! This book serves as your essential companion in navigating the complexities of managing gastritis through delicious, simple-to-prepare meals. Whether you're new to the diagnosis or seeking better symptom management, this cookbook is your ally on the road to enhanced gut health and overall well-being.

Within these pages, you'll discover a diverse array of nourishing recipes crafted specifically to calm and support your stomach. From comforting soups and gentle smoothies to fulfilling main dishes and snacks, each recipe is meticulously designed with your gastritis in mind. Moreover, you'll find invaluable tips, meal-planning strategies, and dietary insights to empower you in making informed nutritional choices.

Remember, effective gastritis management involves not only what you eat but also how you eat. By adopting mindful meal preparation practices and prioritizing the nourishment of your body, you can seize control of your gastritis symptoms and embark on a journey toward digestive wellness. Allow this cookbook to be your trusted companion as you embrace a gastritis-friendly diet and set forth toward a future of improved health and vitality. Here's to relishing the voyage and savoring the delights of happy, healthy eating!

TABLE CONTENT

Introduction

Welcome to the Gastritis Diet Cookbook for Beginners! In this book, you'll discover tasty recipes designed specifically for people with gastritis. We know managing gastritis can be tough, but with the right diet, you can feel better. Inside, you'll find easy-to-make dishes like soothing soups, comforting stews, nourishing smoothies, and light salads—all gentle on your stomach and delicious. But this book is more than recipes; it's a guide to help you understand what foods to eat and avoid to ease your symptoms and promote healing. Whether you're new to gastritis or looking for healthy meal ideas, this cookbook is here to help you cook with confidence and support your digestive health journey. So, let's get cooking and enjoy flavorful, healing meals together!

Chapter 1: Understanding Gastritis

This section delves into the intricacies of gastritis, a common gastrointestinal ailment characterized by inflammation of the stomach lining. It examines the diverse triggers of gastritis, such as bacterial infections, excessive alcohol consumption, prolonged usage of nonsteroidal anti-inflammatory drugs (NSAIDs), and stress. Through detailed discussions and practical examples, readers gain insight into the symptoms and potential complications associated with gastritis, including abdominal discomfort, nausea, vomiting, and even stomach ulcers. Additionally, it explores diagnostic methods, treatment choices, and preventive measures to effectively manage and alleviate gastritis symptoms. This chapter acts as a comprehensive guide for understanding the nature, causes, and management of gastritis, empowering readers to make informed decisions regarding their gastrointestinal health.

What is Gastritis?

Gastritis is a medical condition characterized by inflammation of the stomach lining. This inflammation can present as acute, occurring suddenly and lasting briefly, or chronic, persisting over an extended period.

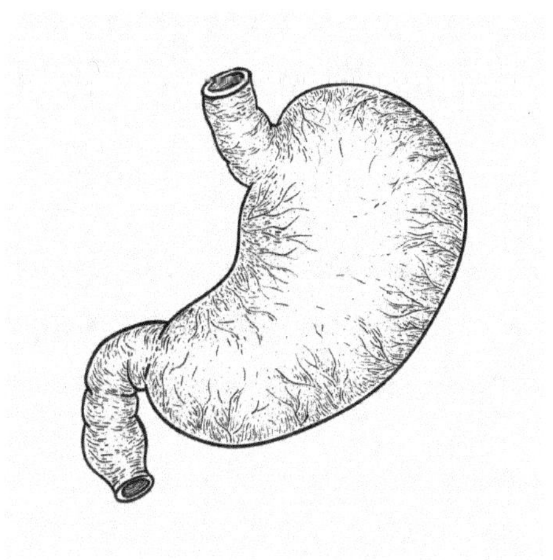

<u>Causes and Symptoms</u>

Gastritis can be caused by various factors, including:

<u>1. Infection with Helicobacter pylori:</u>
This bacterium commonly induces gastritis by infecting the stomach lining and causing inflammation.

<u>2. Regular use of NSAIDs:</u> Nonsteroidal anti-inflammatory drugs (NSAIDs) such as aspirin, ibuprofen, and naproxen can irritate the stomach lining, leading to gastritis.

<u>3. Excessive alcohol consumption:</u> Alcohol can irritate and erode the stomach lining, triggering inflammation.

<u>**4. Stress:**</u> Although stress alone may not directly cause gastritis, it can worsen existing symptoms and exacerbate the condition.

<u>**5. Autoimmune disorders:**</u> In certain cases, the immune system mistakenly attacks the cells of the stomach lining, resulting in gastritis.

Symptoms of gastritis can vary depending on severity and underlying causes but may include:

1. Abdominal discomfort or pain: Ranging from a dull ache to a sharp, stabbing sensation in the upper abdomen.

2. Nausea and vomiting: Some individuals may experience nausea and vomiting, particularly after eating.

3. Indigestion: Gastritis can cause indigestion, including bloating, gas, and a feeling of fullness after meals.

4. Loss of appetite: Some people may experience reduced appetite or early satiety during meals.

5. Black or tarry stools: Severe cases of gastritis may lead to stomach bleeding, resulting in black or tarry stools.

Types of Gastritis

There are several types of gastritis, including:

1. Acute gastritis:

This sudden onset gastritis is typically triggered by irritants like NSAIDs, alcohol, or infections, often resolving with treatment.

2. Chronic gastritis:

Developing gradually and potentially lasting for years, chronic gastritis can result from H. pylori infection, autoimmune disorders, or long-term use of NSAIDs or alcohol.

3. Erosive gastritis: Characterized by erosion of the stomach lining, erosive gastritis can lead to ulcers and bleeding, often associated with

prolonged NSAID use or excessive alcohol consumption.

4. Autoimmune gastritis: In this type, the body's immune system mistakenly attacks the cells of the stomach lining, causing inflammation and mucosal damage.

Understanding the causes, symptoms, and types of gastritis is essential for accurate diagnosis and effective treatment. If gastritis is suspected or symptoms are experienced, consulting a healthcare professional for proper diagnosis and management is crucial.

Chapter 2: Fundamentals of the Gastritis Diet

Gastritis, characterized by inflammation of the stomach lining, brings discomfort like abdominal pain, bloating, and nausea. Understanding the right dietary choices is key to managing symptoms effectively. This chapter delves into the foods to avoid, foods to embrace, and strategies for meal planning to alleviate gastritis symptoms.

Foods to Avoid:

1. Spicy Fare:
Ingredients such as chili powder, black pepper, and hot sauce can exacerbate stomach irritation.

2. Acidic Choices: Citrus fruits, tomatoes, and vinegar can ramp up stomach acid, worsening gastritis discomfort.

3.Fatty Selections: Fried foods, fatty meats, and full-fat dairy products can slow digestion and trigger symptoms.

4 Alcohol: This irritates the stomach lining, leading to increased acid production and inflammation.

5.Caffeine: Beverages like coffee and tea heighten stomach acid production, intensifying symptoms.

6. Carbonated Beverages: These can cause bloating and discomfort for those with gastritis.

7. Processed Foods: Chips, fast food, and packaged snacks are often loaded with unhealthy fats and additives, worsening symptoms.

Foods to Include:

1.Fiber-Rich Options: Fruits, vegetables, whole grains, and legumes support digestion and stomach health.

2. Lean Proteins: Opt for poultry, fish, tofu, and legumes to ease the digestive workload.

3.Probiotic-Rich Foods: Yogurt, kefir, sauerkraut, and kimchi foster a healthy gut microbiome and digestive wellness.

 4.Complex Carbs: Whole grains like brown rice, quinoa, oats, and barley offer sustained energy and digestive support.

5. Fruits: Incorporate bananas, melons, apples, and pears for less stomach irritation.

6.Low-Fat Dairy: Choose skim milk, yogurt, and cheese to reduce saturated fat intake.

Herbal Teas: Indulge in comforting herbal teas such as chamomile, ginger, and peppermint, which possess properties to ease gastritis symptoms and aid digestion.

Meal Planning Tips:

1. Opt for Smaller, More Frequent Meals: Incorporating smaller meals throughout the day can prevent stomach overload and reduce symptoms.

2. Chew Thoroughly: Take your time to thoroughly chew food, facilitating digestion and lessening the stomach's workload.

3. Maintain Hydration: Ensure adequate hydration by drinking ample water daily to support digestive function.

4. Identify Trigger Foods: Steer clear of gastritis-triggering foods and track them in a food diary to eliminate potential irritants.

5. Healthier Cooking Methods: Choose cooking techniques like steaming, baking, grilling, or boiling over frying to cut down on unhealthy fat consumption.

6. Practice Mindful Eating: Cultivate mindful eating habits by listening to your body's hunger and fullness signals, and avoiding rushed or distracted meals.

By adhering to these dietary guidelines and meal planning strategies, you can effectively manage gastritis symptoms and foster stomach well-being. Consulting with a healthcare professional or registered dietitian for personalized dietary advice based on your condition and medical history is crucial.

Chapter 3: Morning Meals - Gastritis Diet Cookbook for Beginners

In this segment of our guide for beginners navigating a gastritis diet, we explore breakfast options tailored to soothe the stomach and offer vital nutrients for a healthy start to the day. Gastritis, characterized by inflammation of the stomach lining, requires mindful dietary selections to alleviate symptoms and promote healing..

1. Nourishing Oatmeal

Oatmeal emerges as a gentle and easily digestible breakfast choice, ideal for individuals with gastritis. This recipe involves cooking rolled oats to a comforting consistency, sweetened with honey or maple syrup for a touch of sweetness. Toppings such as sliced bananas, berries, nuts, seeds, or a sprinkle of cinnamon not only enhance flavor but also deliver nutritional value. Oats are renowned for their soothing properties, making this dish an excellent selection for a gastritis-friendly breakfast.

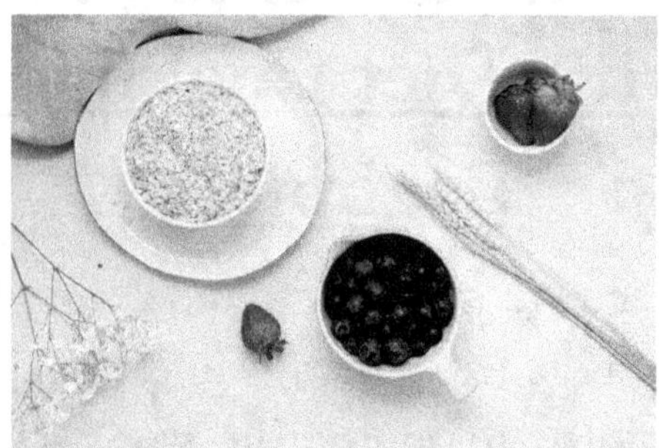

Oatmeal

2. Silky Banana Almond Smoothie

This smoothie presents a creamy fusion of ripe banana, almond milk, almond butter, and vanilla extract. Almonds contribute healthy fats and protein, while bananas offer natural sweetness and potassium, which can help soothe the stomach. This smoothie is gentle on digestion and can be customized with additional ingredients like spinach or oats for added fiber and nutrients.

3. Tofu Scramble with Vegetables

For those embracing a plant-based diet or seeking a protein-packed breakfast, scrambled tofu with vegetables is a fitting choice. Tofu, a versatile ingredient, can be seasoned and cooked to emulate the texture of scrambled eggs. In this recipe, firm tofu is crumbled and cooked with onions, bell peppers, and spinach for a flavorful dish. Turmeric lends color and anti-inflammatory properties, while nutritional yeast provides a cheesy flavor sans dairy. This. the breakfast option is gentle on the stomach and brimming with plant-based goodness.

Each of these breakfast recipes is thoughtfully designed to adhere to a gastritis-friendly diet, prioritizing whole, nourishing ingredients that promote digestive health and minimize discomfort. By integrating these recipes into your morning routine, you can commence your day with delectable and comforting meals that aid in gastritis relief and overall well-being.

Breakfast is often hailed as the most crucial meal of the day, supplying the energy and nutrients needed to kickstart your morning. In this chapter, we introduce three delightful and nutritious breakfast recipes to fuel your day.

1. Comforting Oatmeal

Mild Oatmeal Recipe for Gastritis:

Ingredients:
1 cup of rolled oats
2 cups of water or low-fat milk
1 tablespoon of honey or maple syrup (if desired)
1/2 teaspoon of ground cinnamon (optional)
1/4 cup of mashed banana or applesauce (optional, for sweetness and creaminess)
A pinch of salt

Instructions:
1. In a saucepan, gently boil the water or milk.
2. Add the rolled oats and lower the heat.
3. Cook the oats, stirring occasionally, for 5-7 minutes until desired consistency is reached.

4. Optionally, add honey or maple syrup, mashed banana or applesauce, cinnamon, and a pinch of salt.

5. Allow to cool slightly before serving.

Nutritional Information per Serving:
Calories: ~150
Carbohydrates: ~27g
Protein: ~5g
Fat: ~2.5g
Fiber: ~4g

Tips for Children with Gastritis:
1. Encourage frequent, small meals to avoid stomach irritation.
2. Avoid spicy, acidic, or fatty foods that may trigger symptoms.
3. Choose bland, easily digestible options like oatmeal, rice, bananas, and applesauce.
4. Limit carbonated drinks and caffeine, as they can worsen gastritis.
5. Ensure adequate hydration with water throughout the day to aid digestion.

6. Watch portion sizes to prevent overeating, which strains the stomach.

7. Teach mindful eating practices, such as thorough chewing and eating slowly.

8. Introduce relaxation techniques like deep breathing or gentle yoga to manage stress, which can exacerbate gastritis.

Remember to consult healthcare professionals or dietitians for personalized dietary advice for managing gastritis in children.

2. *Almond Banana Smoothie*

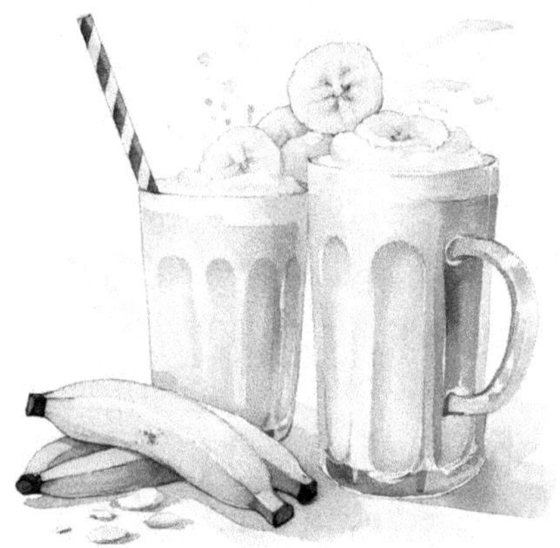

Ingredients:

1 ripe banana
1/2 cup almond milk (or any milk)

2 tablespoons almond butter

1/2 teaspoon vanilla extract

Handful of ice cubes

Steps:

1. Peel banana, place in blender.

2. Add almond milk, almond butter, vanilla extract, and ice cubes.

3. Blend until smooth and creamy.

4. Pour into a glass and serve immediately.

3. Tofu Veggie Scramble

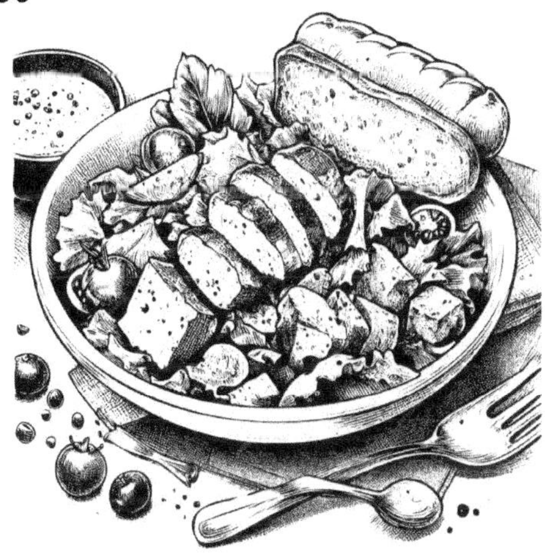

Ingredients:

1 block firm tofu, drained and crumbled

1 tablespoon olive oil

1/2 onion, diced

1 bell pepper, diced

1 cup spinach, chopped

2 tablespoons nutritional yeast

1/2 teaspoon turmeric powder

Salt and pepper to taste

<u>Steps:</u>

1. Heat olive oil in a skillet, sauté onion and bell pepper until soft.

2. Add crumbled tofu, nutritional yeast, turmeric, salt, and pepper. Stir.

3. Cook for 5-7 minutes until tofu is heated and slightly browned.

4. Add spinach, cook 2-3 minutes until wilted.

5. Serve hot, garnish with fresh herbs if desired.

<u>Enjoy these nourishing breakfast ideas to kickstart your day!</u>

Chapter 4: Midday Meal Choices

This section explores a variety of nutritious and delicious lunch options to keep you satisfied and energized throughout your day. Whether you lean towards light and refreshing or hearty and fulfilling, these lunch suggestions have something for everyone.

1. Grilled Chicken Salad

A classic lunch option, the grilled chicken salad provides a balanced blend of protein, healthy fats, and essential nutrients. Begin by grilling seasoned chicken breast to your liking. Then, dice an assortment of fresh vegetables such as lettuce, tomatoes, cucumbers, and bell peppers. Toss everything together with a light vinaigrette dressing for a refreshing and satisfying meal.

2. Quinoa Veggie Bowl

Quinoa veggie bowls are not only tasty but also packed with nutrients. Cook quinoa according to package instructions and set aside. Meanwhile, sauté your favorite vegetables like spinach, bell peppers, zucchini, and cherry tomatoes in olive oil until tender. Combine the cooked quinoa and veggies in a bowl, and top with avocado slices, crumbled feta cheese, and a drizzle of balsamic glaze for extra flavor.

3. Avocado Toast with Poached Egg:

Avocado toast with poached egg is a simple yet fulfilling lunch option that's both nutritious and delicious. Start by toasting whole-grain bread until golden brown. Spread mashed ripe avocado onto the toast and season with salt, pepper, and red pepper flakes for a hint of spice. While that's cooking, poach an egg until the whites are set but the yolk is still runny. Place the poached egg on top of the avocado toast and garnish with chopped cilantro or microgreens for a burst of freshness.

These lunch ideas are not only easy to prepare but also customizable to your taste preferences and dietary needs. Whether you're craving a light salad, a hearty grain bowl, or a simple yet satisfying toast, these recipes are sure to please your palate and keep you fueled for the day ahead.

Chapter 5: Gastritis-Friendly Dinners

In this chapter, we present three recipes suitable for individuals with gastritis. These dishes are not only gentle on the stomach but also full of flavor. Whether you're a novice or an experienced cook seeking fresh ideas, these recipes are guaranteed to please your palate while being kind to your digestive system.

1. Herb-Baked Salmon

Herb-Baked Salmon: A Gastritis-Friendly Delight

In the realm of gastritis-friendly cuisine, herb-baked salmon stands as a beacon of taste and health. This delectable dish not only tantalizes the taste buds but also caters to the dietary needs of kids, making it a star in any gastritis diet cookbook.

Origins: The origins of herb-baked salmon can be traced back to ancient civilizations where fish was a staple in many diets due to its abundance and nutritional benefits. However, the specific recipe for herb-baked salmon emerged more recently, likely in the late 20th century, as people began to explore healthier cooking methods and flavor combinations.

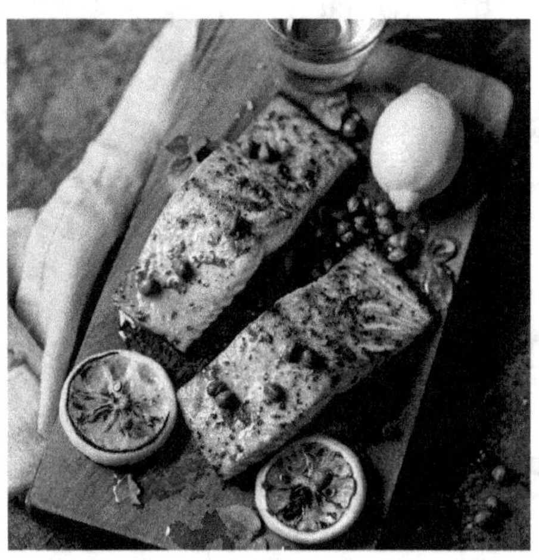

Ingredients: The beauty of herb-baked salmon lies in its simplicity. Key ingredients include fresh salmon filets, a blend of herbs such as dill, parsley, and thyme, garlic, lemon juice, olive oil, salt, and pepper. These wholesome ingredients not only enhance the flavor of the salmon but also contribute to its gastritis-friendly nature.

Preparation: To prepare herb-baked salmon, begin by preheating the oven and lining a baking dish with parchment paper. Next, place the salmon filets on the prepared dish and season them with a mixture of chopped herbs, minced garlic, lemon juice, olive oil, salt, and pepper. Allow the salmon to marinate for a few minutes to absorb the flavors fully. Then, bake the salmon in the oven until it is cooked through and flakes easily with a fork. The result is tender, flavorful salmon infused with the aromatic essence of herbs.

Health Benefits: Herb-baked salmon is not only delicious but also incredibly nutritious, making it an ideal choice for kids following a gastritis diet. Salmon is rich in omega-3 fatty acids, which have anti-inflammatory properties that can help alleviate symptoms of gastritis. Additionally, the herbs used in this dish are packed with antioxidants and vitamins, further boosting its nutritional value.

Beginners-Friendly Appeal:

Newcomers to cooking can find herb-baked salmon to be a delightful first step. With its mild flavor and tender texture, it's an inviting option for those who are hesitant to try new dishes. Moreover, involving beginners in the cooking process can foster excitement and a stronger bond with their meals, leading to a deeper appreciation of the outcome.

Conclusion: Herb-baked salmon is more than just a dish – it's a testament to the intersection of flavor, health, and simplicity. In the context of a gastritis diet cookbook for beginners it shines as a versatile and nutritious option that the whole family can enjoy. With its rich history and undeniable appeal, herb-baked salmon is sure to remain a beloved favorite for generations to come.

2. Vegetable Stir-Fry with Brown Rice

<u>**Historical Overview:**</u>

For centuries, vegetable stir-fry with brown rice has been a beloved dish in Asian cuisine, celebrated for its delightful taste, vivid colors, and healthful qualities. It gained popularity among those embracing a gastritis-friendly diet due to its blend of fresh vegetables and whole grains, providing vital nutrients while being gentle on the stomach.

Ingredients:

1. <u>Brown rice:</u> This fiber-rich whole grain is a nutritional cornerstone, brimming with vitamins and minerals.

2. <u>Assorted vegetables:</u> Opt for a colorful mix like bell peppers, broccoli, carrots, snap peas, and mushrooms to enrich both flavor and nutrients.

3. <u>Olive oil:</u> A heart-healthy addition that lends richness without causing stomach irritation.

4. Garlic and ginger: These aromatic elements not only enhance taste but also boast anti-inflammatory properties, advantageous for gastritis sufferers.

5. Low-sodium soy sauce: Adding depth of flavor without raising sodium levels, is crucial for managing gastritis symptoms.

6. Optional protein: Tofu, chicken, shrimp, or lean beef can provide protein, but it's wise to choose lean cuts and cook them gently to avoid aggravating gastritis.

Nutritional Benefits:

Vegetable stir-fry with brown rice is a nutrient powerhouse, offering essential vitamins, minerals, fiber, and antioxidants. Brown rice, a complex carbohydrate source, sustains energy and supports digestive health. The medley of colorful vegetables contributes vitamins A, C, and K, along with fiber, promoting gut health and aiding digestion. Including protein, whether from tofu or lean meats, helps balance the meal and fosters a feeling of fullness.

1. Opt for low-acid vegetables: Select non-citrus options like bell peppers, carrots, and broccoli to minimize stomach lining irritation.

2. Cook vegetables until tender: Softening vegetables through stir-frying or steaming eases digestion, reducing potential discomfort for gastritis sufferers.

3. Moderate spicy ingredients: While garlic and ginger enhance flavor, excessive spice can worsen gastritis symptoms, so use them judiciously.

4. Control portion sizes: Avoid overeating, even of healthy foods, as it can trigger gastritis symptoms; practicing portion control is key.

5. Maintain hydration: Adequate water intake supports digestion and hydration, particularly crucial for those managing gastritis.

Incorporating vegetable stir-fry with brown rice into a gastritis diet cookbook for beginners offers a delicious, nourishing option that supports digestive well-being.

3. Turkey Meatballs in Tomato Sauce
Title: Turkey Meatballs in Tomato Sauce

Historical Context:

Turkey meatballs have been a culinary tradition for centuries, originating in the Mediterranean and evolving into a versatile dish enjoyed worldwide. Ground turkey, herbs, and spices, simmered in tomato sauce, offer a timeless and satisfying meal.

Ingredients:

1 lb ground turkey

1/4 cup breadcrumbs (gluten-free if preferred)

1/4 cup grated Parmesan cheese

1 egg, lightly beaten

2 cloves garlic, minced

1 tsp dried oregano

1 tsp dried basil

1/2 tsp salt

1/4 tsp black pepper

2 tbsp olive oil

1 onion, finely chopped

2 cloves garlic, minced

1 (28 oz) can crushed tomatoes

1 tsp dried basil

1 tsp dried oregano

Salt and pepper to taste

Fresh basil leaves for garnish (optional)

Nutrition Facts (per serving):

Calories: 280

Total Fat: 15g

Saturated Fat: 4g

Cholesterol: 120mg

Sodium: 560mg

Total Carbohydrates: 10g

Dietary Fiber: 2g

Sugars: 4g

Protein: 26g

Tips for Beginners on a Gastritis Diet:

1. Choose lean meats like turkey to minimize gastritis symptoms.

2. Opt for gluten-free breadcrumbs if you have gluten sensitivity or celiac disease.

3. Avoid overly spicy or hot ingredients in the sauce to prevent stomach irritation.

4. Ensure meatballs are thoroughly cooked to eliminate harmful bacteria.

5. Pair meatballs with gentle sides like steamed veggies or rice for a balanced meal.

Enjoy this delicious and stomach-friendly recipe as part of your gastritis diet journey!

Chapter 6: Gastritis-Friendly Snacks and Sides dish options

In this section, we introduce three snack and side dish ideas suitable for those with gastritis. These recipes are simple, nutritious, and gentle on the stomach, making them great choices for those starting on a gastritis diet.

1. Yogurt Berry Parfait

Historical Background:

Dating back centuries, Yogurt Berry Parfait originates from the Mediterranean, where yogurt has been a dietary staple since ancient times. The dish gained widespread popularity in the late 20th century in Western cultures as a convenient and nutritious option for breakfast or snacks. Its adaptability and health benefits have made it a preferred choice among health-conscious individuals and those managing gastritis.

Ingredients:

1. we of Greek yogurt (plain or flavored)
2. 1/2 cup of assorted fresh berries (such as strawberries, blueberries, raspberries)
3. 1/4 cup of granola

Optional: Honey or maple syrup for sweetness

Preparation Time:

Preparation of Yogurt Berry Parfait is quick and effortless, typically taking only 5-10 minutes, making it suitable for any time of day.

Nutritional Information:

Yogurt Berry Parfait is not only delicious but also rich in essential nutrients beneficial for overall health and digestion. Here's a nutritional breakdown per serving:

1. Calories: Approximately 200-250

2. Protein: 10-15 grams

3.Carbohydrates: 25-30 grams

3.Fat: 5-10 grams

4. Fiber: 3-5 grams

5. Vitamins and minerals: Abundant in calcium, vitamin C, and antioxidants from the berries.

Gastritis Diet Tips for Beginners:

For individuals following a gastritis-friendly diet or those with sensitive digestive systems, consider the following adjustments for a more suitable Yogurt Berry Parfait:

1. Opt for Low-Fat Yogurt: Choose low-fat or fat-free Greek yogurt to reduce fat intake, which can help prevent gastritis flare-ups.

2. Avoid Added Sugars: Steer clear of flavored yogurts with added sugars. Instead, sweeten your parfait naturally with a drizzle of honey or maple syrup, or opt for plain yogurt sweetened with stevia or a sugar substitute.

3. _Choose Granola Wisely:_ Select granola varieties carefully, as some store-bought options may be high in fat and sugar. Look for low-sugar options or consider making your own using oats, nuts, and seeds.

4. _Be Mindful of Acidic Fruits:_ While berries are generally well-tolerated, individuals with gastritis may need to limit or avoid highly acidic fruits like citrus fruits (e.g., oranges, lemons) in their parfait.

5. _Practice Portion Control:_ Enjoy Yogurt Berry Parfait in moderate portions to prevent overeating, which can aggravate gastritis symptoms. Pay attention to your body's signals and stop eating if discomfort arises.

Following these tips, beginners can craft a delectable and gastritis-friendly Yogurt Berry Parfait that supports digestive health and overall well-being as part of a balanced diet.

2. : *A Gastritis-Friendly Option*

Historical Background:

Hummus, originating from ancient Egypt, is a beloved Middle Eastern dip enjoyed worldwide. It's crafted from chickpeas, tahini, lemon juice, garlic, and olive oil, offering a rich history and versatile flavor profile.

Ingredients:

1. 1 can (15 oz) chickpeas, drained and rinsed
2. 1/4 cup tahini
3. 2 cloves garlic, finely chopped
4. 2 tablespoons lemon juice
5. 2 tablespoons olive oil
6. Salt, to taste
7. Assorted veggies for dipping (carrots, cucumber, bell peppers, cherry tomatoes, etc.)

Preparation Time:

This hummus and veggie plate takes approximately 10 minutes to prepare.

Nutritional Value:

Hummus (per serving - about 2 tablespoons):
Calories: 70
Total Fat: 4g
Saturated Fat: 0.5g
Sodium: 115mg
Total Carbohydrates: 7g
Dietary Fiber: 2g
Protein: 2g

Gastritis Diet Tips:

1. Hummus is generally well-tolerated by those with gastritis due to its gentle ingredients. However, monitor your sensitivity to garlic and citrus.

2. Choose whole grain or gluten-free crackers if raw veggies worsen symptoms.

3. Moderate olive oil in the hummus if fatty foods cause discomfort.

4. Experiment with steamed or roasted veggies if raw ones are problematic.

5. Enhance flavor with herbs like parsley or cilantro, which are gentle on the stomach.

Enjoy this hummus and veggie plate as a nutritious, gastritis-friendly snack or light meal.

3. Roasted Sweet Potato Wedges

Roasted sweet potato wedges boast a lengthy heritage dating back centuries. Originating in the Americas, sweet potatoes were cultivated thousands of years ago in Central and South America, where indigenous communities likely roasted them as a primary cooking method.

In the 16th century, European exploration, spearheaded by figures like Christopher Columbus, introduced sweet potatoes to Europe. Their popularity soared, eventually becoming a culinary staple worldwide.

The emergence of roasting sweet potatoes in wedges gained traction in the United States, where these tubers have been a dietary mainstay for generations.

This method's appeal lies in its simplicity: slicing sweet potatoes into wedges and roasting them with seasoning and oil became a favored side dish.

In recent times, roasted sweet potato wedges have surged in popularity, thanks to their delectable taste, adaptability, and nutritional benefits. Often touted as a healthier substitute for traditional french fries, they offer a delightful blend of sweet and savory flavors. Moreover, they are rich in essential nutrients such as vitamins A and C, fiber, and antioxidants, appealing to health-conscious individuals.

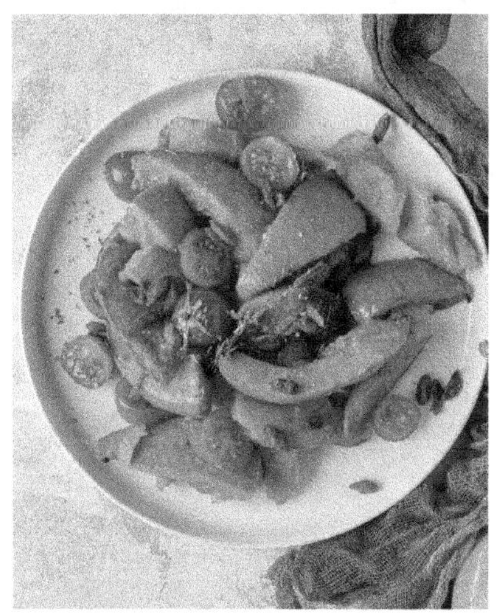

Ingredients:

Sweet potatoes, cut into wedges
Olive oil
Garlic powder
- Paprika
- Salt and pepper

Instructions:

1. Preheat the oven to 400°F (200°C) and line a baking sheet.
2. Toss sweet potato wedges with oil, garlic powder, paprika, salt, and pepper.
3. Spread wedges on the baking sheet.
4. Bake for 25-30 minutes until golden and crispy.
5. Serve hot as a tasty snack or side dish.

These snack and side dish options offer a range of flavors and textures while being gentle on the stomach. Customize them with your favorite ingredients and spices, and enjoy without worry!

Chapter 7: Gastritis-Friendly Desserts

Enjoying desserts while managing gastritis doesn't have to be complicated. Here are three delicious options designed to be gentle on the stomach yet full of flavor. These recipes are perfect for those starting on a gastritis diet and are guaranteed to fulfill your sweet cravings without causing discomfort.

1. Mixed Berry Smoothie Bowl

The mixed berry smoothie bowl has an intriguing backstory. It emerged as a twist on the classic smoothie, which gained favor in health circles during the late 20th century as people became more health-conscious.

In the early 2000s, it gained momentum alongside the rising popularity of acai bowls from Brazil. These bowls typically featured a blend of acai berries with other fruits, topped with granola, nuts, and fresh fruit.

The mixed berry smoothie bowl took inspiration from this trend, incorporating a mix of berries like strawberries, blueberries, raspberries, and blackberries. This blend offered a rich source of antioxidants, vitamins, and fiber, making it both nutritious and flavorful.

By the 2010s, it became a fixture in health-focused cafes and eateries worldwide, thanks to its appealing appearance and customizable toppings, making it a hit on social media platforms like Instagram.

Today, the mixed berry smoothie bowl remains a favorite among health-conscious individuals and food enthusiasts, continually adapting with new variations and ingredient combinations to cater to diverse tastes and dietary needs.

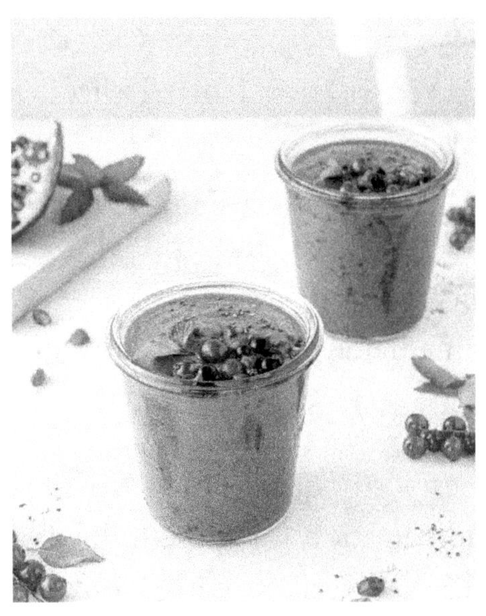

Ingredients:

1. Frozen mixed berries (e.g., strawberries, blueberries,raspberries)
2. Frozen banana, sliced
3. Plain Greek yogurt
4. Optional: Honey or maple syrup
5. Toppings: sliced fresh fruit, granola, nuts, seeds, shredded coconut

Instructions:

1. Blend frozen berries, banana slices, and Greek yogurt until smooth.
2. Add honey or maple syrup if desired.
3. Pour into a bowl and top with fresh fruit, granola, nuts, seeds, or coconut.
4. Serve immediately for a refreshing and nutritious dessert.

A mixed berry smoothie bowl can be a delicious and nutritious option for those following a gastritis diet. Here's a recipe with some nutritional information and tips:

Nutritional Information:

1.Calories: Approximately 250-300 per serving (depending on specific ingredients and portion sizes)

2.Protein: 10-15 grams

3.Fiber: 5-8 grams Healthy fats from almonds and chia seeds

1. Choose ripe, soft fruits like bananas and berries, which are easier to digest.

2. Cinnamon Baked Apples

Cinnamon Baked Apples have long been a cherished dessert, particularly during autumn and winter. They're crafted by coring apples, filling them with a blend of cinnamon, sugar, and occasionally nuts or raisins, then baking until tender. Here's an abridged history:

Origins : Baked apples boast a rich heritage spanning cultures worldwide. The pairing of apples and cinnamon likely traces back to Europe, where both ingredients were plentiful.

Traditional Dish: In the United States, baked apples gained popularity during the colonial period, owing to the abundance of apple orchards and settlers' culinary ingenuity.

Evolution : Over time, the baked apple recipe has transformed, with various regions and families incorporating unique touches. Some variations include oats or breadcrumbs in the filling, while others introduce butter or caramel for added decadence.

Modern Variations: Today, cinnamon-baked apples retain their timeless appeal, valued not just for their delicious taste but also for their simplicity and comforting warmth. They're often served with a scoop of vanilla ice cream or whipped cream for an extra indulgent finish.

Whether enjoyed as a cozy dessert on a crisp evening or as a sweet conclusion to a festive feast, cinnamon-baked apples continue to captivate palates worldwide.

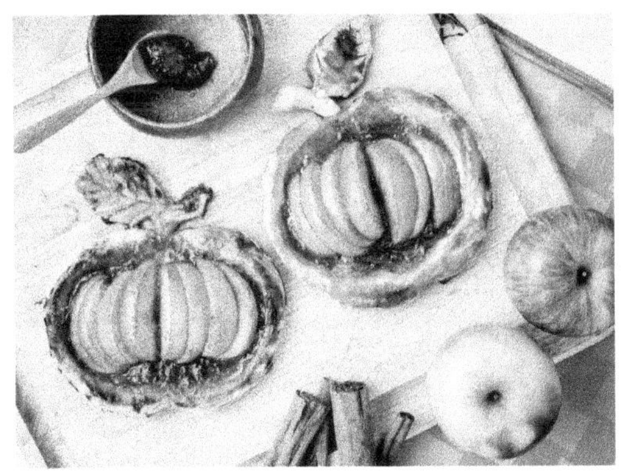

Ingredients:

Apples, cored and sliced

Cinnamon

Optional: Honey or maple syrup

Lemon juice

Optional: Oats

Instructions:

1. Preheat the oven to 375°F (190°C) and grease a baking dish.
2. Arrange apple slices in the dish.
3. Drizzle with lemon juice to prevent browning.
4. Sprinkle cinnamon and drizzle honey or maple syrup if desired.
5. Optional: Add oats for texture.
6. Bake for 20-25 minutes until tender and caramelized.
7. Serve hot for a comforting dessert.

Nutritional Info (per serving, excluding honey/maple syrup and nuts):
  Calories: 95
  Carbs: 25g
  Fiber: 4g
  Sugars: 19g
  Fat: 0g
  Protein: 0g

Gastritis Diet Tips:

1. _Apple Choice_: Opt for sweeter varieties like Fuji or Gala.

2. _Sweetener Control_: Consider skipping honey/maple syrup to avoid symptoms.
3.Portion Management: Stick to smaller servings.

4. _Cinnamon Monitoring_: Start with a small amount to gauge tolerance.

5. _Nuts in Moderation_: Nuts provide healthy fats and protein but can trigger symptoms in some individuals.

3. Vanilla Chia Seed Pudding

Vanilla chia seed pudding has its roots in ancient civilizations like the Aztecs and Mayans, who valued chia seeds for their energy-boosting qualities. As modern health trends evolved, chia seeds became a popular ingredient among health enthusiasts. Vanilla chia seed pudding emerged as a tasty and nutritious way to incorporate these tiny superfoods into everyday diets. By mixing chia seeds with vanilla extract and a liquid such as almond milk, the mixture is left to thicken overnight, resulting in a creamy pudding-like consistency. This versatile dish can be enjoyed as a breakfast, snack, or dessert, offering a rich source of fiber, omega-3 fatty acids, and protein. Today, it continues to be a favorite among those embracing healthy eating habits.

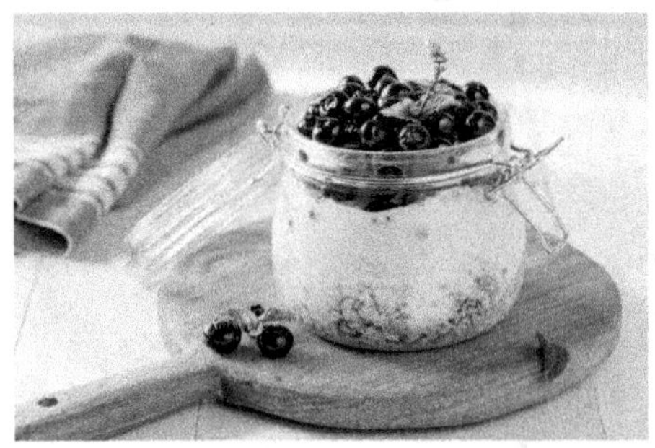

Ingredients:

- 1/4 cup chia seeds

- 1 cup almond milk (or any non-dairy milk)

- 1 teaspoon pure vanilla extract

- 1 tablespoon maple syrup (optional, can be left out for less sweetness)

- 5 minutes (plus at least 2 hours chilling time)

Nutrition Facts (per serving):

Calories: About 150

Protein: Around 4 grams

Fat: Roughly 9 grams

Carbs: Approximately 12 grams

Fiber: About 9 grams

Helpful Tips:

1. _Gentle Mixing_ : Stir the ingredients gently to prevent breaking the chia seeds. Let it sit for a few minutes after stirring.

2. _Adjust Sweetness:_ Customize sweetness to your liking, considering dietary needs. Maple syrup can be skipped or replaced with a suitable sweetener.

3. Consistency: Adjust pudding thickness by varying chia seeds or milk amounts.

4. Flavor Options: Try different flavors like cocoa powder, cinnamon, or fruit purees, ensuring they align with your gastritis diet.

5. Chilling Time: Chill for at least 2 hours or overnight for best results in thickening.

6. Storage: Keep leftovers in an airtight container in the fridge for 3-4 days, stirring it before serving.

Enjoy this soothing and nutritious vanilla chia seed pudding as part of your gastritis-friendly diet!

These dessert recipes provide a tasty way to enjoy sweets while adhering to a gastritis diet. Feel free to customize it with different fruits and toppings. Enjoy these guilt-free treats and indulge in dessert worry-free!

Chapter 8: Soothing Beverages for Gastritis Relief

In this section, we delve into comforting beverage options tailored to alleviate symptoms of gastritis. From gentle herbal concoctions to nourishing smoothies, these recipes are ideal for newcomers seeking comfort and relief.

1. Ginger Infusion

Ginger infusion has a rich history dating back centuries, originating in Southeast Asia where it was valued for its medicinal properties. It was widely used in ancient Chinese, Indian, and Arabic cultures to address various health concerns. As trade routes expanded, ginger made its way to Europe, where it became important in both culinary and medicinal practices during the Middle Ages.

By the 17th century, ginger had become highly sought-after in Europe, leading to the establishment of trade routes with Asia and the Caribbean. The British East India Company played a key role in spreading ginger globally, promoting its cultivation in colonies like Jamaica and India.

In the 18th and 19th centuries, ginger became popular in European and American kitchens for cooking, baking, and making beverages. Ginger beer and ginger ale became favorite non-alcoholic drinks, and ginger-infused teas gained recognition for potential health benefits.

Today, ginger infusion remains popular as a refreshing beverage with possible health advantages. It's known for aiding digestion, relieving nausea, reducing inflammation, and boosting the immune system, appealing to both traditional herbal remedy enthusiasts and modern wellness seekers.

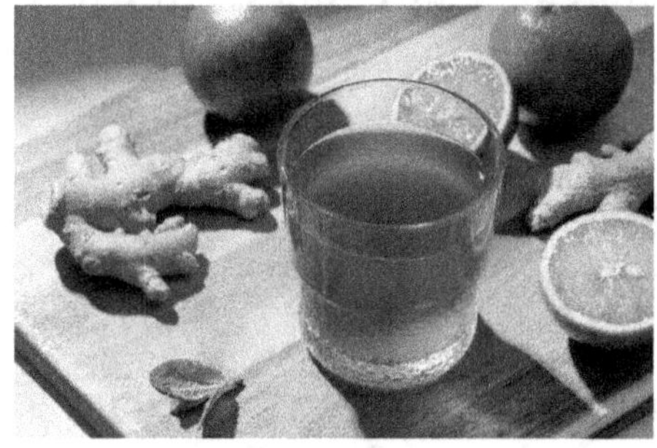

Ingredients:

1. Fresh ginger root, thinly sliced or grated
2. Water
3. Lemon juice (optional)
4. Honey or maple syrup (optional)

Instructions:

1. Bring water to a gentle simmer in a saucepan.
2. Add thinly sliced or grated ginger root to the simmering water.
3. Let the ginger steep for 5-10 minutes, adjusting to taste.
4. Strain the ginger tea into cups and enhance with lemon juice or sweeteners if desired.
5. Serve warm and enjoy the calming and anti-inflammatory benefits of ginger infusion.

Preparation Time:5 minutes

Nutritional Value: Low in calories, rich in antioxidants, and possessing anti-inflammatory properties

Suggestions:

1. Opt for fresh ginger root to maximize flavor and health advantages.

2. Adjust the ginger quantity to suit your taste and sensitivity levels, as it may be overpowering for some.

3. Enhance taste and soothing effects by adding a hint of honey or lemon.

4. Consume the infusion warm for optimal relief, especially during gastritis flare-ups.

5. Explore incorporating other herbs or spices like mint or cinnamon for diverse flavors and additional digestive aid.

2. Herbal Brews

For centuries, herbal brews have been a cherished tradition across various cultures worldwide. Originating from civilizations like the Egyptians, Greeks, and Chinese, these brews evolved into teas, infusions, and decoctions, offering unique flavors and health benefits.

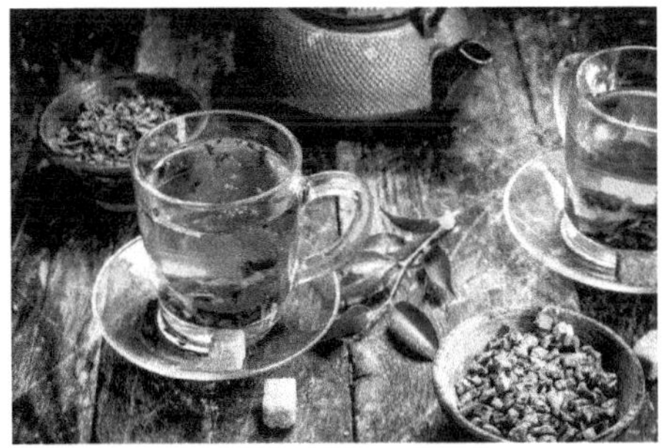

Ingredients for Herbal Brews:

1. Chamomile: Known for its calming effects, chamomile aids digestion and promotes relaxation.

2. Peppermint: Valued for its refreshing taste, peppermint relieves indigestion and nausea.

3. Ginger: With its anti-inflammatory properties, ginger aids digestion and reduces inflammation.

4. Licorice Root: Adding sweetness, licorice root supports gastrointestinal health.

5. Marshmallow Root: Soothing inflammation, marshmallow root aids digestive comfort.

Preparation Time:

Preparation time varies, typically taking 5-10 minutes to steep herbs in hot water. However, some brews may require longer steeping or additional methods like decoction or cold brewing.

Nutritional Value:

While not rich in nutrients, herbal brews offer health benefits through phytochemicals and antioxidants. Chamomile aids sleep and reduces inflammation, peppermint aids digestion, and ginger alleviates nausea and improves circulation.

Tips for Gastritis Diet Cookbook for Beginners:

1. Opt for Soothing Herbs: Choose calming, anti-inflammatory herbs like chamomile, ginger, and licorice root to ease gastritis symptoms.

2. Avoid Acidity: Steer clear of acidic foods like citrus fruits and tomatoes, which can worsen gastritis and irritate the stomach.

3. Experiment with Flavors: Mix herbs and spices to create diverse, palate-pleasing brews tailored to your tastes.

4. Stay Hydrated: Drink plenty of water to support digestion, using herbal brews as a delicious hydration option.

5. Listen to Your Body: Pay attention to how your body reacts to different brews, avoiding ingredients that worsen symptoms.

3. Nourishing Smoothie

The inception of nourishing smoothies coincides with the growing health consciousness of the late 20th century. During the 1970s and 80s, the surge in the health food movement spurred an interest in natural and nutritious foods. Smoothies emerged as a convenient and flavorful solution to incorporate various fruits, vegetables, and wholesome ingredients into a single refreshing beverage.

While the term "smoothie" was coined in the 1960s, it wasn't until the 1990s that it gained widespread popularity. As health and fitness trends continued to rise, smoothie bars and cafes became increasingly common in cities worldwide, offering a diverse range of nutritious blends.

Initially, smoothies primarily featured fruits such as bananas, berries, and mangoes, often paired with yogurt or juice for creaminess. However, as people became more adventurous with their recipes, vegetables like spinach, kale, and avocado found their way into the blender, providing an additional dose of vitamins and minerals.

The proliferation of social media and the internet further democratized smoothie recipes, making them more accessible to a broader audience. Food bloggers and wellness influencers shared their favorite blends, inspiring others to experiment in their kitchens. Today, people of all ages and backgrounds enjoy nourishing smoothies as a quick breakfast option, a post-workout replenishment, or a flavorful means to incorporate extra greens into their diet.

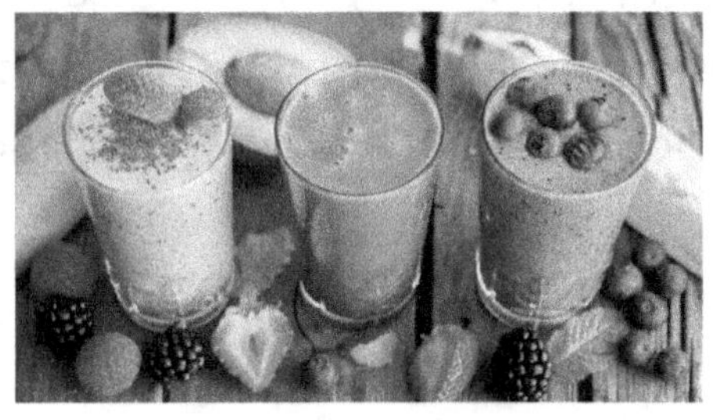

Ingredients:

- 1 cup of plain low-fat yogurt (or a non-dairy alternative)
- 1 ripe banana
- 1/2 cup of cooked, peeled, and cooled sweet potato
- 1/2 cup of fresh or frozen blueberries
- 1 tablespoon of honey (optional, depending on taste)
- -1/2 teaspoon of ground ginger (optional, for its anti-inflammatory properties)
- 1/2 cup of water or coconut water (adjust thickness to preference)

*Preparation Time:*Around 5 minutes

Nutritional Value: This smoothie is packed with fiber, potassium, antioxidants, and probiotics. It offers essential vitamins and minerals while being gentle on the stomach, ideal for individuals with gastritis. The exact nutritional content may vary based on the ingredients used.

Tips for a Gastritis Diet:

1. Opt for ripe bananas to aid digestion.
2. Cooked and cooled sweet potatoes are milder on the stomach compared to raw ones.
3. Choose plain yogurt without added sugars or flavors to prevent irritation.
4. Use honey sparingly if tolerated, for sweetness.
5. Ginger can help calm the stomach and promote digestion; however, if it's too potent, you can omit it.
6. Blend the smoothie until it's smooth and easily drinkable to any digestion issues.

These beverage recipes provide soothing relief and digestive aid for individuals managing gastritis symptoms. Integrate these drinks into your daily regimen to support gut health and overall wellness. Experiment with different ingredients and flavors to discover your preferred combinations. Enjoy these beverages as part of your gastritis-friendly diet and appreciate the comfort they bring.

Chapter 9: Strategies for Dining Out and Social Events

In this chapter of the "Beginner's Guide to the Gastritis Diet," we explore tactics for adhering to your gastritis-friendly eating plan while dining out or participating in social gatherings. Managing restaurant menus and communal meals can pose challenges, but with the right strategies, you can make wise choices and relish your meals without worsening gastritis symptoms.

Making Informed Decisions at Restaurants

1. Research and Plan in Advance : Before dining out, take time to explore restaurants offering gastritis-friendly options. Look for menus featuring lean proteins, cooked vegetables, and whole grains. Many restaurants now provide nutritional details online to help you make informed decisions.

2. _Customize Your Order:_ Don't hesitate to request modifications to suit your dietary requirements. Ask for grilled or steamed dishes instead of fried options, and request sauces and dressings on the side to control portions and avoid triggers like spicy or acidic ingredients.

3. _Choose Simple Preparations:_ Opt for dishes prepared simply, with minimal added fats, spices, and sauces. Grilled or baked proteins like chicken or fish, paired with steamed vegetables or a plain baked potato, can be safe and satisfying choices.

4. _Mindful Portion Control_ : Restaurant portions are often larger than home servings. Consider sharing an entrée with a companion or asking for a half portion to prevent overeating and undue strain on your digestive system.

5. _Stay Hydrated:_ Opt for water or herbal tea over sugary sodas or alcoholic drinks, which can irritate the stomach lining. Adequate fluid intake can help soothe inflammation and promote healthy digestion.

Bringing Your Gastritis-Friendly Dish

1. Plan Ahead: If attending a potluck or social gathering with buffet-style food, bring a dish aligned with your gastritis diet to ensure a safe option for yourself amidst other offerings.

2. Choose Simple Recipes : Select easy-to-prepare and transport recipes like salads, roasted vegetables, or lean protein dishes. Avoid ingredients known to trigger gastritis symptoms, such as citrus fruits, tomatoes, and spicy peppers.

3. Communicate with Hosts : Inform hosts about your dietary restrictions beforehand, so they can accommodate your needs or suggest suitable dishes. Most hosts will appreciate your proactive approach and be happy to help.

4. Label Your Dish : Clearly label your gastritis-friendly dish with ingredients, especially if it contains common allergens or triggers. This ensures other guests are aware of any dietary restrictions and can enjoy your contribution safely.

By following these strategies, you can confidently navigate dining out and social events while supporting your meals gastritis diet and overall well-being. With a bit of planning and preparation, you can savor delicious and socialize with friends and family without compromising your health.

Gastritis Diet Cookbook for beginners: 30-Day Meal Planner

Welcome to the Gastritis Diet Cookbook for beginners! This month-long meal guide is crafted to help ease gastritis symptoms while offering tasty and nourishing dishes. By adhering to this plan, you'll explore an array of flavorful recipes that are gentle on your stomach and support digestive wellness.

<u>*Week 1: Gentle Beginning*</u>

Day 1:

- **<u>Breakfast</u>:** Warm oats topped with banana slices and a drizzle of honey
- **<u>Lunch</u>:** Grilled chicken breast served with steamed carrots and quinoa
- **<u>Dinner</u>:** Baked salmon paired with roasted asparagus and brown rice

Day 2:

- **<u>Breakfast</u>:** Greek yogurt mixed with berries and a sprinkle of granola
- **<u>Lunch</u>:** Spinach and turkey wrap with avocado in a whole grain tortilla
- **<u>Dinner</u>:** Tofu and vegetable stir-fry with brown rice

Day 3:

- **<u>Breakfast</u>:** Pineapple and spinach smoothie blended with banana and almond milk

- **Lunch:** Quinoa salad with cucumber, cherry tomatoes, and crumbled feta
- **Dinner:** Cod filet baked alongside steamed broccoli and sweet potato

Day 6:.

- **Breakfast:** Cottage cheese topped with peach slices and a drizzle of honey
- **Lunch:** Quinoa and black bean salad tossed with diced bell peppers and lime dressing
- **Dinner:** Baked chicken thighs served with roasted Brussels sprouts and quinoa

Day 7:

- **Breakfast:** Overnight oats made with almond milk, chia seeds, and mixed berries
- **Lunch:** Tuna salad lettuce wraps filled with cucumber and tomato
- **Dinner:** Stir-fried tofu with bell peppers and snap peas, served over brown rice

Day 8:

- **Breakfast:** Whole grain pancakes served with Greek yogurt and sliced strawberries
- **Lunch:** Grilled vegetable and chicken skewers paired with quinoa salad
- **Dinner:** Baked tilapia alongside sautéed spinach and mashed sweet potato

Day 9:

- **Breakfast:** Smoothie bowl topped with banana slices, granola, and honey
- **Lunch:** Vegetable and lentil soup enjoyed with a side of mixed green salad
- **Dinner:** Turkey chili topped with diced avocado, served with whole grain cornbread

Day 10:

- **Breakfast:** Scrambled eggs with diced tomatoes, served on whole grain toast

- **Lunch:** Greek salad topped with grilled chicken breast and lemon vinaigrette
- **Dinner:** Baked cod served with roasted Brussels sprouts and quinoa pilaf.

Continue with this meal plan format for the remaining days, gradually introducing new recipes and variations to maintain a balanced and enjoyable diet. Emphasize lean proteins, whole grains, abundant fruits and vegetables, and healthy fats in each meal. Encourage hydration by drinking water throughout the day and avoiding trigger foods that could worsen gastritis symptoms. Enjoy your journey towards improved digestive health with the Gastritis Diet Cookbook for beginners!

Conclusion

Congratulations on completing the "Beginner's Guide to the Gastritis Diet"! You've gained valuable insights into managing gastritis through diet and learned to prepare nourishing meals that support digestive health.

Reflecting on Your Journey

Take pride in your progress toward better health. Whether new to managing gastritis or seeking new strategies, this guide has provided a solid foundation for success.

Embracing a Gastritis-Friendly Lifestyle

Remember, managing gastritis involves not just what you eat but also mindful eating, stress management, and physical activity.

Continuing Your Gastritis Diet Journey

Experiment with new recipes and seek support from friends, family, and healthcare professionals who understand your needs.

Moving Forward with Confidence

Armed with knowledge from this guide, move forward confidently in managing gastritis and embracing a vibrant life.

Thank you for joining us on this journey to a gastritis-friendly diet. Here's to your continued success and well-being!

9 798326 451262